Healthcare & Medical Apps
(Smartphone Apps are Revolutionizing Healthcare)

Author: Paul E. Love

Copyright 2018 Paul E. Love

Other Books by the Author:

The Employer's Payroll Question and Answer Book 2018
Rescue Me: Animals in Need
The Drone Question and Answer Book
Anatomy of a Google Sheets Project
The Sports Dictionary
Find an IT Job
The Volunteer's Guide

CONTENTS

Introduction

There's a quiet revolution (or maybe "evolution" is more accurate) going on in the healthcare industry.

Over the last ten years over 250,000 mobile healthcare apps have appeared on the scene – and that's only the beginning. According to estimates from Zion Market Research the market for mHealth (mobile health) apps will top $100 billion worldwide in 2018. With smartphones and tablets becoming an essential part of our lives it makes sense to provide apps for those devices that can help organize your medical records, monitor your health, alert you to a possible medical problem, and help connect you to a healthcare professional.

So how do smartphones function as medical devices? The cameras, microphones, and other sensors built into smartphones are improving all the time and can already be used to help diagnose certain illnesses The microphone for example, can be used to help detect asthma and COPD (Chronic Obstructive Pulmonary Disorder). There are also apps that use the camera and flash to diagnose blood disorders such as iron and hemoglobin deficiency. Smartphones can even by used to detect conditions such as osteoporosis by using the phone's motion sensor.

Doctors and medical researchers are also turning to smartphone technology as an efficient way to handle electronic health data. Having patients collect data relating to their medical condition by using a smartphone app can make it much easier for a physician to form a diagnosis and to follow up on the effectiveness of the treatment the patient is undergoing. And that same data collected from many different patients can be a gold mine for medical research personnel, providing them with a massive database of clinical information never available before.

This book covers just a few of the many different types of mobile health apps available on the market today. Dozens more (including many that offer new and more advanced technology) are being added everyday. Consider this book a sampler – and, if you're interested in building a mobile health care app yourself, you'll also find some introductory information about building your own app. Welcome to the future of healthcare!

Overview

What are the basic types of medical and healthcare apps on the market?
Here are the general categories of mobile medical/healthcare apps:
- Healthy living apps (fitness and exercise, diet monitoring, cardio monitoring and healthy nutrition)
- Women's health apps (for pregnancy, baby feeding, and infant care)
- Weight loss apps (weight loss tracking, diets, exercises)
- Medication tracking (tracking proper time intervals and dosages)
- Symptom tracking and self-diagnosis
- Chronic medical condition monitoring (diabetes, cancer, heart problems)
- Mental health apps
- Emergency/urgent care
- Medical records tracking
- Patient medical education
- Anatomy/Physiology learning apps
- Medical billing and coding
- Healthcare provider locating and consultation
- Doctor on demand apps

What are the benefits of using a healthcare app?
- Studies have shown that patients recording information using a healthcare app tend to provide more honest and reliable information than when talking face-to-face with their doctor. Part of the reason may be that they can take their time, plan what they want to say, and make additions and corrections at their own pace.
- A healthcare app that can alert you to a medical problem before it gets really serious can make a big difference in keeping you healthy (and catching a problem early can also make a significant difference in your healthcare costs).
- Apps which allow you to carry out a virtual doctor visit can also save you money compared to a in-person visit to a physician. Employers are even starting to encourage employees to take advantage of these kind of apps too, hoping that a quick online visit can help reduce the number of employee sick days. (Interesting note: According to an article in Computerworld,

almost 1 in 6 doctor visits were already virtual visits in 2014).

What makes smartphones a good platform for health-related apps?

Current smartphones (and some tablets) can act as the platform for different healthcare apps primarily because they have a variety of embedded sensors. Apple iPhones sensors include a barometer, accelerometer, touch ID fingerprint sensor, proximity sensor, a 3-axis gyro, and an ambient light sensor. Samsung Galaxy Android phones include a pressure sensor, fingerprint sensor, iris sensor, accelerometer, barometer, gyro sensor, proximity sensor, and an RGB light sensor.

General Medical/Healthcare Apps

WebMD
Probably the best-known health care app, WebMD offers a variety of features including:

- Symptom Checker – Select the part of your body that you think is affected and choose your symptoms and WebMD will provide information regarding possible conditions or issues.
- Conditions – Read medically reviewed information about specific medical conditions including causes, symptoms and treatments.
- Drugs and Treatments – Read about different drugs, vitamins and supplements including proper usage and possible side effects.
- First Aid – WebMD offers a quick guide to all types of situations requiring first aid, from bug bites to broken bones.
- Pill Identification – Identify prescription and over-the-counter medicines by pill shape, color and imprint.
- Local Health Listings – Find your closest pharmacy, physician or hospital based on your current location. You can also search by city, state and zip code.

Doctor on Demand
Doctor On Demand makes instant access to health care a reality. Patients can download the app to their smartphone, tablet or desktop computer and instantly Video Visit from home with a board-certified physician for pediatric, psychological, lactation needs and more. No appointments, and no dragging a sick child to the pediatrician. The first Video Visit is free, and after that, the cost is $40. Some insurance providers even cover the fee.

MyChart
Patients can download MyChart on either the App Store or Google Play and use it to access health data from previous in-office visits to healthcare providers. Viewable data includes test results, immunizations, medication, and health conditions indicated by the provider. MyChart also allows a patient to confirm appointments, pay their healthcare bills, and upload patient-generated data such as fitness metrics from a wearable health device. Through the app, patients can also message their providers and confirm/schedule appointments.

Apple Health
Apple Health can track everything from your steps and calorie intake to your blood pressure and fiber intake (with the help of some third-party apps and devices). It can even store details of your medical history and your medical records. Apple Health also works with a number of popular fitness trackers, particularly its cousin, the Apple Watch.

Google Fit
Google Fit is either already installed on your Android phone or you can download it from the Google Playstore. It works automatically – as long as you have your phone on you it will keep track of your steps as you walk, run or cycle (or you can add activities manually). You can also display various statistics (such as time, steps, distance or calories) while you're in the middle of an activity. In addition, a number of wearable fitness trackers can be synced to Google Fit if you don't want to have to carry your phone with you.

Fitness Builder
Fitness Builder Includes over 1,000 workouts along with more than 7,000 images and videos to help guide your workouts. You can track your results, record body measurements and chart your progress.

Lifesum (iOS)
Designed to help you achieve a healthy lifestyle, Lifesum features a general health quiz, a workout plan, healthy meal recipes, body monitoring and a meal tracker.

The Johnson & Johnson Office 7-minute Workout
This app is designed for people who are short on time but want to improve their physical fitness. You can choose a workout intensity level that matches your ability and the app will help coach you through each step of the workout.

Health Tap (free)
Health Tap provides free guidance, advice and health tips from over 100,000 doctors whenever you need it from a library of over 6 billion answers to different healthcare questions. Or send your own particular question and get personalized responses quickly from doctors in 141 specialties. You can also pay for an actual consult via text or audio or video chat at any time, day or night.

Atmosphere Relaxing Sounds
The app has over 100 different relaxing sounds you can choose to help you relax and get to sleep. Options include city sounds, forest sounds and beach sounds.

MyNoise
myNoise is another app to help you get to sleep. You can mix sounds from the app with other sounds on your phone – for example you can play music while you listen to ocean waves.

Test Your Hearing (free from EpsilonZero)
This simple hearing test app produces different sounds or tones at varying frequencies to help you test your hearing acuity. You also have to identify the difference (softer, louder) in sounds at different frequencies.

Depression CBT Self-Help Guide (free – Excel At Life)
Stress can lead to depression and this app attempts to help you control the stress in your life. The app includes a depression severity test along with articles, emotion training and relaxation audio clips, a cognitive diary and a motivational points system to help you learn about depression and how to deal with it. The goal is to teach you how to manage stress and engage in self-care behaviors that can reduce your symptoms and improve your mood. It also contains a complete cognitive-behavior therapy (CBT) guide to help you learn to practice positive thinking.

WikiMed
WikiMed is an offline encyclopedic medical dictionary offering a comprehensive collection of health-related articles, including content on diseases, medications, anatomy and sanitation. WikiMed does take up a hefty 1.1 gigabyte, so make sure you have enough storage space available to install it (if you're short of space you can try WikiMed Light instead).

Fooducate
You can use this app to scan food product bar codes right in the grocery store and the app will display the nutrition grade (A-D). You can also track your food intake, calories and exercise level and you can connect to the Fooducate online community to share questions, tips and general information.

S Health

A free app built into Samsung phones, this self-maintenance app features a pedometer, calorie counter, exercise tracker and sleep diary. You can also sync with third-party blood pressure monitors and glucose meters — all over Bluetooth.

iTriage

iTriage was designed by two emergency room physicians to answer two questions: "What's wrong with me?" and "Where can I go for help?". The app provides short, easily understood definitions of symptoms, diseases and procedures, along with a list of medications, including descriptions, dosages and possible side effects. Once a user has determined a possible cause for his symptoms he can use the app's "System-to-Provider" pathway to locate appropriate healthcare or medical providers in the area (ranging from pharmacies to urgent care locations to individual physicians). Provider information may include distance, consumer ratings, years of experience, gender, wait times and languages spoken. (free for iPhone and Android).

HemaApp

HemaApp uses a smartphone's camera to screen for anemia without the need for a blood draw or an expensive machine to non-invasively measure hemoglobin counts. HemaApp illuminates a patient's finger using the smartphone's camera flash and analyzes the color of the blood to estimate hemoglobin concentration. The user simple places a finger over the camera and triggers the flash. A video is generated from the data acquired from the flash and is translated into an estimate of hemoglobin concentration in grams/deciliter units (g/dl).

BiliScreen

BiliScreen is designed to test for pancreatic cancer and other diseases by having the user take a number of selfies and then scanning those images. It uses computer vision algorithms and machine learning tools to detect increased bilirubin levels in a person's sclera (the white part of the eye). Jaundice (a yellowing of the skin and eyes due to elevated levels of bilirubin) is one of the earliest signs of pancreatic cancer (and other diseases). Pancreatic cancer has one of the worst survival rates partially because it isn't usually detected until the cancer is well advanced; BiliScreen may help indicate at-risk patients much earlier.

Apps to Help You Understand Medical Terms

Medical Dictionary – Healthcare Terminology
This app is a directory of medical terms and concepts containing around 180,000 terms covering different branches of medicine. It provides definitions and brief descriptions of different diseases and many of the items include audio and pictures. You can search for concepts by title and content and you can also add your own notes. (free for Android and iOS).

Medical Terminology
A free Android app covering often used medical terms and their definitions. Includes the ability to search for terms using an alphabetical index.

Anatomy & Physiology in a Flash!
This multi-media app from the Skyscape provides reference information and flashcards for anyone looking to develop a basic understanding of the functions and structures of the human body. It includes 15 sections organized by body system and color-coded and each section contains tips and quiz questions to test the user's understanding of the material in that section. There are over 250 full color flash cards covering the body's structures and the cards can be bookmarked for additional study later. Users can also create custom quizzes to improve areas of weakness based on answered questions. The app also provides a question of the day . Note: In-app purchases must be made in order to access all questions.

Apps for Organizing Your Medical Records

Track My Medical Records

This free Android app allows you to keep a list of immunizations, allergies, medical conditions and other information, as well as charting blood pressure and blood sugar data for you and your family. Your data is backed up to the Internet and transferred by means of an encrypted connection to protect your privacy. You can also go to www.freehealthtrack.com in order to access your information from your desktop computer or other non-Android device.

My Medical

My Medical is an iOS app and costs $19.99 (a free trial is available). For twenty dollars you get a standard record tracking app that lets you keep a list of your medical conditions, procedures and drugs, but you also get additional details about exactly what each type of medication is for, along with side effects, dosages and frequency. In addition you can track lab and test results using the app's charting feature and you can easily transfer records from one system to another.

iBlueButton

iBlueButton is a record keeper for Medicare beneficiaries. The idea behind it is that people will save money on healthcare procedures by keeping their medical records all in one place because Medicare beneficiaries tend to see a higher number of care providers who don't necessarily talk to each other.

Apps to Help with Medical Bills

<u>Better</u>

Better is an app for filing out-of-network health insurance claims. You pay your bill, then take a photo of the bill and send it to Better's team and they handle the rest, including determining your eligibility (not all policies pay for out-of-network care) and following up with your health insurance company to make sure your claim gets paid.

<u>Simplee</u>

Simplee's mobile app aims to help people manage and pay all their family's medical bills through a smartphone. Key features of the Simplee app include getting a detailed breakdown of medical bills, confirmation of deductible or other insurance coverage, and the ability to pay by credit, debit, or FSA/HSA card.

<u>CakeHealth</u>

CakeHealth is designed to help you manage your health care bills. The service connects to major health insurance providers and then pulls in your claims, deductibles, and other data so you can see how your insurance has covered you and know which services are covered or require co-payment. Other features include billing alerts in case you may have been overcharged on a medical bill.

Apps for Finding Fair Prices

GoodRx

GoodRx helps you find the best deal on prescription drugs. You enter your zip code and your prescription and GoodRx searches nearby pharmacies to locate the lowest cost for your prescription. It also lets you know about any discounts, coupons, or other assistance available, and provides information about Medicare coverage. Once you choose a pharmacy you'll also get a coupon you can present to the pharmacist (be aware though, that drug discounts can seldom be used with insurance). Having GoodRx available means you can look up information about a prescription as soon as your doctor suggests it; and if the drug isn't covered by your insurance or you can't afford it you can ask right then if there's a comparable alternative.

Healthcare Bluebook

This app asks for your zip code and then it lists the fair price in your area for medical, dental and vision procedures, lab work, X-rays, medications and even doctor visits. The maker also suggests that you can use the information Healthcare Bluebook delivers to negotiate lower prices when you receive a bill with charges that are well above the fair price shown by the app.

Apps to Reduce Stress

Fabulous
Fabulous takes an all-encompassing approach to building better habits through incremental lifestyle changes. Developed in the behavioral economics lab at Duke University, Fabulous includes methods backed by scientific research. You can choose one of four habits to focus on (sleeping better, feeling more energized, improving concentration and focus, or losing weight) and it provides tools to help you including alarms, reminders to buy certain groceries, recipes, short workouts and meditations.

Calm
Calm incorporates a wide range of activities proven to reduce stress. Relaxation techniques built into the app include:
- Progressive muscle relaxation – in this technique you focus on slowly tensing and then relaxing each muscle group, which helps you develop the ability to relax your muscles when you tense up due to stress.
- Visualization - In this technique, you form mental images to take yourself on a visual journey to a peaceful, calming place or situation. For best results you should involve as many senses as possible, including sight, sound, smell and touch. For example picture yourself at the beach, listening to the sound of the waves washing ashore, the smell of salt water and the warmth of the sun on your face.
- Fictional stories – Stories with sound and visualizations designed to relax you and help you sleep.

I Love Hue
This app is a game that combines art with puzzles and a calming aesthetic. You move tiles to arrange them in chromatic order. The result is a mental challenge alongside soothing phrases, music and colors. This incorporates the benefits of calming imagery, mantras and audio along with a bit of art therapy, which has also been shown to reduce stress.

Apps to Help You Keep Up with Healthcare News

Medscape MedPulse App
This app is updated daily with Medscape's published medical news articles, trending medical news and selected blog content. You can customize the news announcements to include just those that are relevant to your interests and MedPulse also allows you to share articles to your social media accounts. The app is free for both Android and iOS users, although you do have to sign up with a Medscape account (www.medscape.com/public/medpulseapp).

Medical News Online
Free Android app from Medibilim that delivers the latest healthcare and medical news from various medical journals, podcasts, online articles and other sources. You can filter the results by category such as:
* Oncology
* Cardiology
* Allergy
* Immunology
* Genetics
* Pediatrics
* Surgery
* Nutrition and Diet

NEJM This Week
The New England Journal of Medicine (NEJM) is one of the most respected medical journals and the NEJM This Week app covers the latest medical research published in the journal in the last seven days, including review articles and perspectives.

Apps to Let You Take Part in Medical Research

WebMD Pregnancy App
This popular app includes a study platform built on Apple's ResearchKit technology and has connected researchers with a highly engaged group of study participants. Over the first nine months of the program, over 2,000 participants from all 50 states were enrolled into the study and completed over 100,000 daily measurements of activity, sleep, heart rate and blood pressure.

EpiWatch
EpiWatch works with your iPhone to collect research material on adults with epilepsy. The goal is to use the data collected to help create a seizure detecting app to provide advance warning of a seizure. You can use the app to take surveys, make entries in a daily journal and participate in other activities which (with your permission) will be shared with researchers.

StopCOPD
StopCOPD lets you take part in a research study focused on lung health, with the goal of gaining a better understanding of COPD. Participants can complete tasks and submit surveys from the app, and it can record and track your health data using Apple's ResearchKit framework. You don't have to have been diagnosed with COPD to take part in the study – current and former smokers are welcome, along with those with a family history of respiratory disease.

Autism and Beyond
The goal of this study is to test new video technology that can analyze a child's emotions and behavior. Hopefully, the end result will be a screening and evaluation process which can supply parents with tools to better understand their child, as well as providing assistance if needed. Note: Data from participants can be sent with or without video.

DreamLab
DreamLab is part of the DRUGS (Drug Repositioning Using Grids of Smartphones) cancer research project. Researchers at Imperial College London are working with the Vodaphone Foundation to recruit people to donate the power of their smartphones to run an app that can help carry out research overnight. The project hopes to harness

the processing power of thousands of smartphones (while the phones are charging overnight or otherwise not in use) to analyze huge volumes of data. While a participant's phone is sitting overnight charging the app runs for six hours, downloading a data packet about 5 MB in size and running millions of calculations before uploading the results and clearing the data. Note: DreamLab has already been used by researchers in Australia to analyze data for pancreatic cancer.

Pregnancy and Baby Care Apps

BabyCenter
Includes a pregnancy tracker, baby calendar, due date calculator, name finder, contraction timer, feeding guide and baby care advice.

WebMD Pregnancy App
Offers a variety of features including:
- Checklists such as what to buy for your pregnancy and what to take to the hospital.
- Photos that cover each stage of pregnancy so you can see week by week what changes are taking place in your body.
- Questions that you may want to ask your doctor (and the ability to store the answers).
- Special content for women expecting twins or triplets.
- Access to the WebMD pregnancy community.

The Guy's Guide to the Delivery Room
This app helps prepare new dads for what's going to happen in the delivery room. It includes a guide to the different stages of labor they can expect to see and how to recognize each stage, how to make the mother-to-be more comfortable, and simple explanations of terms such as C-section and episiotomy.

Today's Parent My Family
A comprehensive baby care app. New mothers can find tips and information on everything from dealing with postpartum depression to weaning your child from a pacifier to dealing with potty training. It also has a "storybook" feature which allows you to combine photos and videos of your baby in order to create a digital scrapbook.

Baby Bundle
Baby Bundle allows you to track all of your baby's day to day activities: nap times, feeding times, pooping, and so forth. It also includes features such as a vaccination guide, a breastfeeding timer, and a parenting guide. And for $2.99 Baby Bundle can also be turned into a baby monitor.

Weight Management Apps

Lose It!
Winner of the Surgeon General's Healthy Apps Challenge, Lose It! is a valuable app for anyone trying to lose weight through dieting and/or exercise. When you download the app you have to enter your age, gender, height, weight, your target weight and the rate at which you would like to lose weight (from one half pound to two pounds per week). Once you've done that, Lose It! displays a recommended daily caloric intake.

The program works as a food and exercise journal, helping you to monitor your eating habits. You stay on track by scanning a food product's bar code or searching for it in the food database to find it's caloric content. You can also "add exercise" by type and duration from a list, which includes everything from badminton to bowling. The app then subtracts the calories burned from the daily calories you've consumed. Graphs show you the progress you've made, while alerts let you know if you've forgotten to log food or exercise. You can also share your progress with others via Facebook and Twitter.

Lose It! Is free for both iPhone and Android.

Fooducate
Fooducate provides you with the actual nutritional value of foods you buy or are considering buying. Simply scan a food's bar code or search for it in Fooducate's database, and the app assigns the food a "health grade," which can range from a healthy A to a dismal D. If you don't like a product's rating, Fooducate offers healthier alternatives. (free for both iPhone and Android).

Digital Therapeutics Apps

What are Digital Therapeutics Apps?
Digital therapeutics are a new category of apps that help treat diseases by attempting to modify patient behavior and by providing remote monitoring to improve patients' long-term health outcomes. Depending on the disease, they can encourage patients to stick to diet and exercise programs or help them adhere to drug intake regimes. Digital therapeutics apps implement treatment programs tailored to specific ailments, particularly major chronic diseases like mental illness, diabetes, heart disease, high blood pressure, obesity, and pulmonary diseases like COPD.

Because patient behavior is crucial in preventing and limiting the severity of these types of life-threatening illnesses, these digital health programs combined with human advice and interaction can often make a significant difference in a patient's health. They can be tailored to specific patients and can act as a personal health coach.

How important are digital therapeutics apps?
Chronic diseases account for over 85 percent of all health care costs in the United States. If digital therapeutics can help reduce the costs involved with these diseases they could be a major boon to healthcare professionals.

What's driving the explosion in digital therapeutics apps?
Mobile apps are can be delivered on a massive scale at very low cost and by preventing the onset or progression of different diseases they can potentially save insurers billions of dollars.

Are there different categories of digital therapy apps?
Digital therapy apps are generally split into two categories: those that focus on a single disease and those that focus on general health and wellness. Examples of the first category include:
- **Hello Heart** – Hello Heart is a blood pressure app. You can add new blood pressure readings, display a graph of previous readings, maintain a list of your medications, get feedback on your blood pressure readings and tips on beneficial lifestyle modifications.
- **Omada** - Omada is a digital health management program designed to help prevent diabetes. Users have access to online

coaches who can suggest lifestyle choices to help avoid diabetes. The app helps you to track your meals, your physical activity and your weight.

Apps in the second category (general health and wellness) include **MyFitness Pal**, and **Noom**.

Which type of digital therapeutic apps are more effective?

Apps focused on a single disease are more effective simply because most people don't feel any impetus to spend time on a general wellness app. If you're already dealing with a specific condition you're already motivated to explore options such as digital therapeutics.

Are there any potential problems with single disease digital therapeutic apps?

A weakness in single disease applications is that there may be more than one underlying cause affecting people dealing with a given disease. Often there are both mental and physical aspects involved and an app that deals with just the physical part of the problem offers only a partial approach to therapy.

Pharmaceutical Apps

Pharmapedia
Pharmapedia is a free offline app that provides you with information on generic drugs (including dosages and indications), along with a list of brands of medicine with prices, available forms, and alternate brands.

Pharmaceutical Dictionary (Candle Light Apps)
Pharmaceutical Dictionary is a free medical app that provides information about almost all drugs used for medication: uses, dosage, how to take, side effects, precautions, drug interactions, missed dose effects and storage.

Pocket Pharmacist (Danike Inc.)
Pocket Pharmacist is an iOS app that features summarized drug information on the top 1,700+ medications in the United States. The drug summaries have been written by licensed pharmacists and are written without the use of technical jargon. In addition to extensive information about each drug, users can also add their own notes.

Disease and Disorder Reference Apps

Disorder & Diseases Dictionary
A free offline app containing a list of medical diseases and disorders that provides information about symptoms, treatment, risk factors, possible complications, related drugs and home remedies. It can be used to look up symptoms and treatments and for self-diagnosis. (free Android app by ufostudio).

Diseases Dictionary Offline 2017
Free, offline dictionary app from Le Duy for iOS. The app contains information on all major diseases and disorders including symptoms, causes and treatment, as well as a guide to medical terminology and prescription drugs.

IDdx: Infectious Disease
This app allows you to search for a disease that fits a certain description and lists any infectious diseases that could relate to that profile. Currently, you can research more than 250 illnesses by 39 epidemiological factors and 16 world regions. IDdx also displays pictures for diagnostics and support for emergency situations.

Apps for Kids

Buster Baxter: Lung Defender

This app was developed by PBS Kids and uses the character "Buster Baxter" from the kids' TV show *Arthur* to teach children about asthma and common triggers. It includes games along with other educational material to help kids to better understand how to live with asthma.

Monster Heart Medic

Monster Heart Medic teaches children about the cardiovascular system The app also offers tips on staying healthy.

Napoleon Bone Apart

Teaches kids about the bones of the human skeletal system in simple, easy-to-understand terms.

A Heart Pumping Adventure

The Human Body Detectives venture into the circulatory system to learn more about the heart, blood and how the circulatory system works.

Simply Sayin'

Children's Hospital developed this app to help young patients to better understand medical jargon and what to expect as a patient. It makes use of colorful pictures and sounds to help them learn how to cope with their medical experiences.

Apps for Cancer Patients

Cancer Terms Pro
As a cancer patient you're going to hear a lot of medical terms in the course of your treatment. Cancer Terms Pro will help you decipher the medical jargon. It includes just those terms connected with oncology and cancer treatment so it's specific to cancer patients – no unrelated terminology. (iOS app, available from iTunes for $1.99).

Cancer Dictionary Free
Another app that offers a quick reference to oncology-related medical terms. Cancer Dictionary Free also includes pronunciation guides and synonyms for terms and drugs used to treat cancer. It has a user-friendly interface and works offline. (iOS app, available from iTunes for free).

Belong (Beating Cancer Together)
Provides cancer patients and their families with the ability to locate support groups for every type of cancer. The service is free and according to their website (https://belong.life/) it includes:
- Access to oncologists, radiologists, researchers and nurses who can answer your questions.
- Assistance, tips, and support from a large social network of others with cancer.
- The ability to organize and manage your records on your mobile device and share them with family or medical professionals.
- Access to a clinical trial matching service specific to your particular type of cancer.

Cancer.Net Mobile
Cancer Net Mobile includes features that allow cancer patients to get up-to-date information on more than 120 types of cancer. You can also log and track your treatments, receive advice on how to manage side effects of treatment and connect to links for cancer-related videos, blogs and podcasts. (free for iOS and Android – also available in Spanish).

My Chemo Brain
One of the most common side effects of chemotherapy is temporary memory lapses. This app allows patients to make notes on-the-spot regarding appointments, medications and conversations with medical

personnel. The notes can serve as reminders and can also be emailed to family and friends to keep them updated. (free for iOS and Android).

My Breast Cancer Coach

My Breast Cancer Coach was developed in partnership with breastcancer.org and Genomic Health, a cancer research institution. The app helps patients navigate potential treatment options by providing understandable information. It includes common questions for doctors, links to patient advocacy websites, a glossary of medical terms, and a calendar. Users can also update the included journal, with text, photo, and audio recordings.

CareZone

CareZone allows you to enter reminders and schedules in addition to tracking what medications you have actually taken and when you took them. You can also take a picture of your meds and supplements and CareZone will automatically add their names, dosages and other details so you always have a complete list of your medications. (free for iOS and Android).

Pocket Cancer Care Guide

This free app, developed by the National Coalition for Cancer Survivorship, uses your phone's recording ability to store conversations with your doctors and nurses. There is also a glossary of medical terms and a calendar to help you keep track of your scheduled appointments. Another feature is a list of hundreds of commonly-asked questions and answers that you can browse through to help find answers to your own questions.

Apps for Individuals with Diabetes

Dexcom G6 Continuous Glucose Monitoring
Dexcom's CGM system provides continuous glucose monitoring via your smartphone without finger sticks and calibrations. It alerts the user when glucose levels are rising or falling and the data can be shared with up to five followers. Trend lines displayed on your screen let you know which direction your glucose levels are heading and how fast they're changing. You can also add customizable alerts and alarms. Note: Dexcom G6 has been approved by the FDA to make diabetes treatment decisions without confirmatory finger sticks or calibration.

Diabetes Buddy Lite
Allows you to track the factors that affect blood glucose levels, including your daily carbohydrate intake, water intake, medication and glucose measures.

Glucosio
An app for those with type 1 or 2 diabetes. Glucosio tracks metrics like A1C (the amount of hemoglobin in the blood that has glucose attached to it), ketones, blood pressure, body weight, and cholesterol level. In addition, if you give the app permission it can share your data anonymously with diabetes researchers. Glocosio can also back up your data to Google Drive and export it to a CSV file. More features (such as additional export formats and basal tracking) are currently in the planning stage (free Android app).

Glucool
You can use Glucool to log measurements such as your HbA1c (the hemoglobin component that measures blood glucose). The app uses those measurements to display data concerning your current glucose level.

MyNetDiary PRO: Calorie Counter and Food Diary
A weight-loss app that doubles as a diabetes app. You can track your body weight, body measurements, symptoms, medication usage, blood pressure, A1C, and more. You can also sync all your devices and set up a daily budget for fat, carbs and protein using the app's food database of over 700,000 entries. ($3.99 for Android and iPhone).

Diabetes Tracker with Blood Glucose/Carb Log

This app by MyNetDiary helps you manage type 1 and 2 diabetes as well as prediabetes and gestational diabetes. You can record a variety of input data including physical activity (using the built-in GPS) and foods (using the built-in bar scanner). Diabetes Tracker lets you monitor your water intake, weight, A1C, net carbs, and cholesterol and it can also supply food grades as well as virtual coaching to help you maintain a healthy lifestyle.

Apps for Heart Disease Patients

Instant Heart Rate +

A free app for iPhone and Android that provides a simple way to monitor your heart rate. It measures your pulse using your smartphone's camera feature – you put your finger in front of the camera and the app measures color changes in your finger. The color changes are linked to your pulse so the program's built-in algorithm can build a graph of your heart rate. Premium features that can be purchased include a fitness and fatigue test, workouts and motivational support.

Blood Pressure Monitor – Family Lite

Free app that uses your iPhone or iPad to measure your pulse and graphs the results to show unhealthy blood pressure trends. It also provides you with additional information, such as how medication affects your blood pressure.

PulsePoint

A free app for Android and iPhone that can connect someone with a cardiac emergency to nearby people with CPR training. The app can also provide the location of the nearest automated external defibrillator (if your area is currently covered by the app's database).

Cardiograph

The app uses your device's camera to take pictures of your fingertip and then determine your heart's rhythm. It also stores every measurement you take, so you can compare readings during different times and even at different locations. Multiple profiles can be created and stored on one device, so you can keep track of readings for your whole family.

CardioSmart Heart Explorer

CardioSmart was developed by the American College of Cardiology with the goal of improving patient care. The app's high-resolution graphics and animations make it easier for doctors to discuss common heart problems and treatments with their patients. Your doctor can use the app to pull up a 3-D beating heart and answer questions using the visual display of the heart. You can also look through the graphics to get a better understanding of your heart's anatomy and how it functions.

AliveCor Kardia Mobile

Alivecor's *Kardia Mobile* app (iPhone) allows the user to perform an ECG (Electrocardiography) analysis on him or herself, using a touch sensor slightly larger than a credit card. The device and app are FDA approved and can detect various abnormalities in the way your heart is functioning, including "AF" (Atrial Fibrillation), "PACs" (Premature Atrial Contractions, and "PVCs" (Premature Ventricular Contractions). It can take a reading without the use of wires, patches or gets – just turn on the app, hit "record now" and place your finger on the electrodes on the sensor and you get your ECG results within seconds. Note: Alivecor has also developed a version of the app called "*Kardia Band*" which works with the Apple watch.

Apps for Patients with Eye Problems

Eye Test – Eye Exam (free from healthcare4mobile)
Eye Test checks for some of the most common eye problems including:
- nearsightedness, farsightedness and astigmatism (using a variety of standard eye charts)
- color perception problems
- cataracts
- macular degeneration
- dry eye
- accommodation spasm

Eye Test include 12 eye tests to track how your vision is doing and 8 eye health quizzes to check your knowledge of the most common vision problems.

EyeNetra
An inexpensive visual acuity tester, for mobile eye diagnostics or vision screenings.

Welch Allyn iExaminer Adapter and Ophthalmoscope
Welch Allyn's iExaminer app and accompanying ophthalmoscope device is designed to make it easier to detect conditions like retinal detachment or glaucoma. The ophthalmoscope device plugs into most smartphones and the accompanying app allows users to email or print the pictures provided by the ophthalmoscope or to store them in a patient file.

Apps for Pets

ASPCA Mobile App
A free app for Android and iOS, the ASPCA mobile app stores your pet's health records, delivers the latest and most relevant news about pets and animal welfare and provides instructions on how to take care of pets in case of a natural disaster.

PetTech PetSaver App
The PetSaver app includes step-by-step instructions for CPR, first aid, and daily health care information for dogs and cats. You can also access a comprehensive list of poisonous items that can be hazardous to your pets. The items are organized by category (Plants, Household Items & Food) and each one includes a description, full-color picture, signs and symptoms and what actions to take if your pet ingests that item. The first aid section contains step-by-step instructions for each type of emergency with pictures and an audio file narrated by Thom Somes (the president of Pet Tech) so that you can listen and follow along with it. In the Essentials Section there are instructions for collecting urine and stool samples, how to restrain and muzzle, how to check your pet's vital signs (breathing rate, pulse, and temperature), what to do in an emergency situation and how to transport an injured pet.

Gibi Pet Locator
Gibi, the pet GPS tracking service, helps pet parents find their four-legged family member with the touch of a button on their smartphone. Pet owners get their pet's accurate location in near real time from anywhere through their Internet connected smartphone.

Apps for Doctors & Medical Personnel

Epocrates
One of the most widely used medical apps, Epocrates is available for both iOS and Android. Doctors use the app to look up drug information and interactions, find providers for consults and referrals and to calculate patient measurements such as BMI (Body Mass Index). Epocrates and the majority of its content is free, although additional information such as alternative medications and lab guides can be purchased for $174.99 per year.

Medscape
Medscape (by WebMD) is a medical reference tool for both iOS and Android. It includes a disease reference guide, drug information and current medical news. Medscape is free but you do have to sign up for a (free) account, which you can do through the app.

MDCalc
MDCalc is a free clinical decision tool that's available for both iOS and Android. It includes over 350 decision tools based on content provided by physicians and medical experts covering more than 150 disease states in 35 specialty areas. According to the MDCalc website, over one million healthcare providers in close to 200 countries make use of the app every day.

Doximity
A free social network for doctors, Doximity has both iOS and Android versions. The app (which Doximity claims is used by 70% of U.S. physicians) allows the user to communicate with other doctors, follow news and trends in medicine, send HIPAA-secure faxes, and browse jobs and salaries. You do have to register and join the network but membership is free.

Prognosis
Prognosis is a free app that allows you to test your diagnostic ability with over 600 simulated clinical case scenarios (with new ones added weekly). Each case has a short, in-depth analysis of the diagnostic process, followed by an up-to-date discussion on the specific condition involved. The cases cover over 30 specialties and each one is reviewed by volunteer specialists who make sure that each scenario is accurate and clinically relevant.

Touch Surgery

Touch Surgery (free for iOS and Android) is an interactive surgical simulator that guides you through a variety of operations. You can:
* Learn operations step-by-step in training mode
* Experience realistic surgical environments with state of the art 3D graphics
* Track your results as a surgeon
* Build a personalized library of surgical procedures
* Learn new techniques
* Use the spy glass feature to identify and learn about the instruments, tissues, muscles and bones involved in each procedure

iMurmur

iMurmur provides recordings of 20 types of heart murmurs, allowing a physician to match and identify what she or he hears.

Pocket Anatomy

Search through through thousands of high resolution images of anatomical structures. Structures are pinned for identification – you can enter notes next to a pin and bookmark content.

Brainscape

A free flashcard app, Brainscape uses the spaced repetition technique to boost learning speed and retention. You can create your own deck of cards to help in memorizing any area of medical knowledge.

Canopy Medical Translator

This app allows you to look up translations for questions and statements in 15 different languages for every aspect of a physical exam. For most languages you can actually play the translations out loud – plus, if you run into problems, there is also direct access to a translator via a phone call.
Http://try.canopyapps.com/canopy-medical-spanish-amsa/

Radiology 2.0 (free – iOS)

CT (Computed Tomography) scans require considerable training in order to be able to read them correctly. Radiology 2.0 provides an interactive experience in reading CT scans – it uses over 7,000 images to help you learn to interpret CT scans correctly. In addition, each case is followed by extensive discussions to explain what you're seeing and the explanation behind it.

Muscle and Bone Anatomy 3D ($4.99 – iOS)
A nicely animated app, this shows you every muscle, joint and bone in the human body in 3D detail. Each muscle is listed by name, action, origin, insertion, and nerve supply, along with explanatory comments. The app also features seven 3D models that allow you to control and manipulate the major bones and joints, view how the muscles contract and how joints move. There are also embedded videos and photos and short quizzes that help you master the material covered by the app.

Diseases Dictionary
A free Android and iOS app, Diseases Dictionary offers a long list of illnesses and conditions that medical personnel are liable to encounter, along with symptoms and preferred treatments. Users can type in a symptom and a list of possible diseases will appear along with comprehensive information about how to deal with the symptoms and how to prevent the disease.

Symptomia
Symptomia can be a useful tool as a quick reference to more than fifty symptoms, their possible causes, and appropriate diagnosis.

Nursing Essentials
This app turns the RN Pocket Guide into a digital information resource. Nursing Essentials includes sections on CPR, Assessing, Cardiac, Respiratory, Neurological, Pediatrics, and more.

Pill Identifier
Pill Identifier by Drugs.com offers a searchable pill guide that allows the user to identify a particular pill. You can search over 10,000 pills by shape, color, strength and more.

3M Littman Soundbuilder
Littman produces medical grade stethoscopes and Soundbuilder is designed to help students and clinicians improve their skill at using a stethoscope. The app includes 14 lessons that provide practice in identifying key heart sounds through the use of text, a virtual mannequin, dynamic waveforms and a 3D animation of a heart in action.

Gauss Pixel App

The Gauss Pixel App provides doctors and nurses with a way to accurately measure the amount of blood loss in a surgical procedure. After taking a picture of surgical sponges used during a procedure with either an iPad or iPhone, the app accurately computes the amount of blood loss in real-time. Currently nurses usually estimate the blood loss in patients with no exact way to determine that information.

Medical Spanish

Helps medical personnel caring for non-English speaking patients by providing audio of commonly used phrases.

Apps for Hospital Patients

The Mount Sinai Hospital Patient Itinerary App
Mount Sinai is currently piloting an iPad app it developed that gives patients a detailed schedule of their upcoming treatments, procedures, and tests. The goal of the app is to alleviate patient stress by keeping them informed with a real-time snapshot of their clinical care information.

CBORD Patient App
CBORD Patient enables self-service meal ordering using a patient's own device—or any hospital-approved mobile device—connected to CBORD food service and nutrition operations.

FindMyPatient
FindMyPatient provides physicians with a list of patients and their locations in real-time to reduce the need for doctors to print information from hospital terminals or call a ward to find out where a patient has been moved to.

NICHE for Patient + Family
The NICHE app helps prepare older adult patients and their caregivers for the realities of hospitalization and transitions between home, hospitals, and nursing homes.

Togethera
Togethera is a simple image, video, and comment sharing service that allows only those who you have invited via email to see what you have shared. It provides an easy way for patients in the hospital to post updates on their condition and share that information with selected friends, co-workers and family members.

Building a Healthcare or Medical App

Why make a healthcare or medical app?
Mobile health care (mHealth) apps have exploded onto the market with the global increase in smartphone usage and figure to be a major part of health care now and in the future. The availability of a mobile framework for these types of apps has gone hand-in-hand with the movement toward more patient-centric health care. They allow users to take charge of a greater part of their own healthcare and keep track of everything from personal health data to medication dosages, symptom monitoring, and doctor consultation.

What are some of the factors you need to be aware of in creating a healthcare/medical app?
If you decide to build a healthcare app (or have one built), you need to consider:
- What features help make an mHealth app successful?
- How do you protect your intellectual property, the thought, design and construction of your app?
- How do you determine if your app will be subject to regulation by the Food and Drug Administration? What steps do you need to take if it does fall under the oversight of the FDA?
- Will your app meet with the approval of the Federal Trade Commission? Does it make claims that the FTC may decide are unfair or deceptive acts or practices?
- What about data privacy and security? The Health Insurance Portability and Accountability Act (HIPAA) applies to any health-related information, so if your app collects, creates or shares a user's health information you must make sure that data is properly protected.
- And of course, you need to have a well thought out plan for how to market your app – how to get it exposure and how to build your brand.

What features are commonly found in mHealth apps?
Standard mHealth components include:
- Scheduling
- Tracking and monitoring
- Social media Integration
- Prescription descriptions and pricing

- Billing and payments (including the ability to pay online and keep track of invoices and payments)
- Photos
- Reviews

What types of data do mHealth apps track?
mhealth apps track items such as heart rate, blood pressure, pulse, glucose levels and caloric intake.

What features go into the making of a successful mHealth app?
Some of the primary features of a good medical app are:
- Easy to install and dependable to use
- Nice looking, easy to use interface
- Protects and preserves sensitive patient information
- Syncs data across various user devices
- Provides a useful service to people who use the app
- Uses videos, games, quizzes, contests and social media to make the app more interesting
- Designed to allow for updates and additions to the app
- Offers the option for a larger, simpler interface for older users

Any tips for apps designed to teach or instruct?
Use repetition to reinforce knowledge retention and incorporate videos, games and quizzes where appropriate in order to keep users engaged.

What differences are involved with apps for healthcare workers?
Apps for healthcare workers emphasize communication with patients. They're designed to create a close connection between the patient and medical workers by monitoring the patient's status and providing for the exchange of information between the patient and medical personnel.

Which platform should I build my app for (Apple, Android, etc)?
Apple had an advantage for years due to the standards applied to all their different platforms (compared with the lack of uniformity for Android devices) but new programming tools have made it much easier to develop for one platform and then convert to other platforms.

How can I find a developer to create my app?
Here are a few options for locating a mobile health app developer:
- Companies that specialize in healthcare app development:

- Claricode (www.claricode.com)
  - MobileSmith (www.mobilesmith.com) (specializes in hospital apps)
  - Steelwiki
- ThinkMobiles provides a directory of software engineers both here in the U.S. and abroad.

What does it cost to have a healthcare app built for you?

The answer is that it depends on a number of factors such as the complexity of the app you want built, the number of pages or screens you want, and which platforms you want it to work with (iOS, Android, Windows Phone, etc.). In order to get a ballpark figure you can get quotes from different software developers, or if you want a quick estimate, Thinkmobiles (https://thinkmobiles.com/blog/how-much-cost-make-app/) has a cost calculator where you can fill in basic information about your app (platforms, pages, database, CRM integration, payment options, etc.) and they will contact you with a price quote.

What programming languages are used to write healthcare apps?

If you're writing an app to run on Apple products (iOS platform) the app will be developed in either Objective-C or Swift – if you're writing an app to run on Android devices it will be probably be programmed in Java.

What if I want to develop an app for both Apple and Android devices but don't know how to code?

You have a number of alternatives if you want to develop an app for Apple and Android at the same time and don't know Objective-C, Swift or Java. For example, both Appcelerator and Adobe's PhoneGap/Cordova/Ionic let you develop in Javascript – then an intermediate layer translates the Javascript code into Objective-C or Java (or other languages). Note: You still distribute via Google Play for Android apps and for-pay in the Apple App Store for iOS apps.

How can I build my own healthcare app without programming?

The easiest way is to find a website that offers a customizable framework that is already designed for creating healthcare apps. For relatively simple, straight-forward apps there are a number of services that may be able to help you develop your app including:

- Appy Pie is a cloud-based do-it-yourself mobile app builder tool that allows users without programming skills to create an app for almost any platform and publish it. Just choose a theme and drag and drop pages onto a smartphone template to create your own mobile app online. Once it's complete, you receive an HTML5-based hybrid app that works with all platforms, including iOS, Android, and Windows. You have the ability to send push notifications, insert ads, see live analytics, and track location with GPS. You can also integrate social media feeds, blogs, websites, audio, radio, and more. You can also insert custom code and embed iframes. Plans start at free with ads and go up to $50 per month.

- AppMachine – Another online app builder, AppMachine lets you design and build native apps for both Android and iOS. You use a drag and drop interface to combine building blocks to create your app. Available building blocks include text, photos, and video, as well as links to Facebook, Twitter or online stores. AppMachine also allows you to scan a website for key content that can be transferred over into your app.

- Good Barber provides a platform to build iPhone and Android apps. For any of the platforms, you can control every detail of the app without writing any code. Several highly customizable design templates are available to get started. Price: Plans start at $32/month for Android apps and at $96/month for iOS apps.

- DB AppMaker - DB AppMaker is an automation tool that can generate Android and iOS mobile apps from MySQL, PostgreSQL, SQLite, Microsoft SQL Server and Oracle databases. It helps you build native-feeling mobile apps using web technologies like HTML, CSS, and JavaScript. You can generate an app which can be tested with your browser or directly on your mobile device. The generated app is fully customizable and can be opened in other tools for further development. DB AppMaker can also output your app in release mode (requires Android Studio) as an .apk file for publishing to Google Play. Or you can open the generated project in Xcode (requires a Mac computer) to output an .ipa file for publishing to the Apple App Store.

What is "app-wrapping"?

App wrapping generally refers to adding (or wrapping) third party software (particularly security software) to an app after the application has been compiled.

What about testing a new app before it's published?

Any program should be tested as thoroughly as possible before its final release. Testing for a new app should include items such as:

- Do some extensive testing of the portions of your app that are designed to keep the user's health information secure – there can be serious penalties for HIPAA violations.
- Beta testing. There is no better way to find the bugs in an app than letting other people try it out and uncover the things that were overlooked or coded incorrectly. Plus beta testers can often point out missing or confusing items in the instructions or even come up with ideas on how to improve your app.
- What if a phone call or message interrupts your app – will events like that crash the app or will it resume right where it left off?
- Is your app well-behaved? Does it hog memory or slow to a crawl if the user has other apps open?

If I build an Apple or Android app how do I distribute it?
To distribute your Android app through the Google Play Store go to https://play.google.com/apps/publish/signup/ and sign in with your Google account. Then accept the terms and pay a $25 registration fee. To market your iOS app through the iTunes store you need to go to https://developer.apple.com/programs/enroll/, pay a $99 annual fee and sign in using your Apple credentials. Once you're published both Google and Apple take 30% of each of your sales.

Is there an easy way for doctors to create mobile apps for their patients?
There are several options that allow doctors or other medical personnel to create an app without having any programming expertise or having to hire a developer:

- Doctella (www.doctella.com) - provides a platform where medical professionals can create apps specific to their practice and each patient's condition without any coding, make it simpler for doctors to check in on patients outside the office. It's designed to make it easier for healthcare providers to build apps using Apple's CareKit, a software framework for developing health apps. By integrating with HealthKit and other hospital-grade medical devices and sensors present on patients' phones or via the cloud, patients can choose to share their information with doctors via Doctella to automatically track reported outcomes, vitals, and actions, exercise routines, pain monitoring and prescriptions. Through Doctella CarePrograms, this information is analyzed to create the context for alerts and

reminders that are shared with the patient, caregiver, and providers.
- AppMaker.com (https://www.appmakr.com/doctors/) - AppMaker for doctors allows you to create your own customized app by modifying their existing framework to add the particular features you want. Include office hours, insurance accepted, directions, contact information, patient reminders, preventative health care tips – whatever items you decide to add. You can also upload PDF copies of your office's patient medical history forms so patients can fill out the forms at home in order to save time when they show up for their appointment. Note: You can create your app for free, but it will include a few "unobtrusive" ads – to remove the ads you have to pay a small monthly fee.

Federal Regulation of Healthcare/Medical Apps

Why is the Food and Drug Administration concerned about healthcare and medical apps?
The FDA wants to apply regulatory control to those apps with a functionality that could pose a risk to a patient's safety if the app were to not function as intended.

What type of apps does the Food & Drug Administration intend to regulate?
The FDA's primary area of concern is mobile health apps that (under FDA rules) can be designated as a "medical device". If a mobile app is intended to be used to perform a medical device function such as diagnosing a disease or other medical condition or providing treatment or prevention of a disease, then the FDA considers that app to be subject to regulation.

What rule covers the FDA definition of a "medical device"?
Section 201(h) of the Federal Food, Drug, and Cosmetic Act defines a medical device:
"... an instrument, apparatus, implement, machine, contrivance, implant, in vitro reagent, or other similar or related article, including any component, part, or accessory, which is intended for use in the diagnosis of disease or other conditions, or in the cure, mitigation, treatment, or prevention of disease, in man or other animals ..."

What types of mobile healthcare apps aren't subject to FDA regulation?
Currently the FDA plans to exercise "enforcement discretion" but not actively regulate healthcare/medical apps that:
* help users manage their disease or medical condition without providing specific treatments or treatment suggestions.
* Provide users with simple tools to track and organize their health information.
* Provide easy access to information related to a patient's medical condition or treatment.
* Help users document, show or communicate potential medical conditions to health care providers.
* Automate simple tasks for health care providers.
* Enable patients or providers to interact with Personal Health Record (PHR) or Electronic Health Record (EHR) systems.

- Transfer, store, convert to a different format, and display medical device data in its original format from a medical device.

The FDA will exercise enforcement discretion regarding these categories of apps because they pose a low risk to users. Basically the FDA will exclude software that doesn't meet the definition of a "medical device" as laid out in the 21st Century Cures Act.

What are the three categories the FDA uses to classify mobile apps?

Mobile healthcare and medical apps are categorized based on their risk profile:
- Class I (general controls; lowest risk)
- Class II (special and general controls)
- Class III (premarket approval required; highest risk)

If an app falls into one of these classes it qualifies as a medical device and must meet all the controls and application requirements for that type of device. For example, a Class II device requires a 510(k) application to be submitted to the FDA prior to the app being released in the commercial market.

What are the two types of apps that qualify as "medical devices"?

Medical device apps are separated into two categories: mobile apps that are intended to be used as an accessory to a regulated medical device and apps that are intended to transform the mobile platform itself into a medical device. For example an app that controls the inflation and deflation of a blood pressure cuff acts as an accessory to a medical device while a smartphone app that works with a blood glucose strip attached to the phone transforms the phone itself into a medical device.

What does HIPAA (the Health Insurance Portability and Accountability Act of 1996) have to do with healthcare apps?

HIPAA was created to protect people's personal health information (phi) and that includes information stored in a healthcare app. Specifically, HIPAA applies to information:
- which is created or received by a covered entity (i.e., a health care provider, health plan or health clearinghouse) and
- which relates to the past, present or future mental or physical health of an individual and
- that identifies the individual

If an app is subject to HIPAA the developer(s) will face a number of obligations that stem from HIPAA's Security Rule. The Security Rule applies to electronic personal health information (ePHI) the same as it does to paper records. Covered entities (and any business associates) must ensure the confidentiality, integrity and availability of all ePHI that the entity creates, receives, maintains or transmits. Failure to comply with HIPAA rules can result in severe penalties.

Note: Data encryption is not mandatory under HIPAA rules – however it will almost always be considered "appropriate" for healthcare apps.

Are there restrictions similar to HIPAA for apps developed in other countries?

Yes, other countries have similar laws that cover the protection of private health care data. For example, mHealth apps developed in Canada are subject to the Personal Information Protection and Electronic Documents Act (PIPEDA) that sets parameters for the administration of personal data by businesses, while mHealth apps developed in Europe fall under EU data protection laws, such as the Data Protection Directive 1995/46/EC (Section 2.1) and the e-Privacy Directive 2002/58/EC (Section 2.2).

CareKit

What is CareKit?
CareKit is an open-source software framework created by Apple for apps that let you better understand and manage your medical conditions.

What do you mean by "a software framework"?
CareKit actually consists of six pre-programmed customizable modules that can be used to track patient care plans, monitor their effect, and share that data with others. The individual modules can be modified and combined in different ways to produce a variety of health care apps.

What are the six modules?
The CareKit modules include:
* Care Card – Can be used to display care plans on the screen of the user's device.
* Symptom and Measurement Tracker – Used to monitor the user's symptoms and track any measurements associated with those symptoms.
* Insights – Displays charts intended to provide the user insight by showing the relationship between treatment and progress.
* Care Plan Store – Stores the data displayed by Care Card.
* Connect - Involve medical care teams and/or family members as partners.
* Document Explorer – Packages the graphs and other information in CareKit's data store for export.

What type of information does Care Card display?
The Care Card module helps the user track the progress of any tasks included in the user's care plan. For example the user might need to take certain medications at specific times, change a dressing, check his or her blood pressure, do some physical therapy, or take a glucose reading. Just about any task that needs to be performed can be displayed and tracked in the Care Card.

What is HealthKit and does it have anything to do with CareKit?
HealthKit is a programming framework created by Apple. It's designed to house healthcare and fitness apps, allow them to work together and collate their data under Apple's Health app. The collected data is then

saved in a database called HealthStore, which can be accessed by
CareKit, providing a built-in data source for CareKIt apps.

What are some examples of apps created with CareKit?
CareKit based apps include:
- One Drop – A diabetes control app, One Drop tracks your food,
  medication intake and activity.
- Glow Nurture - Tracks all the timings that are important during
  pregnancy - due dates, doctor's appointments and so on - and
  lets you log weight changes and symptoms.
- Glow Baby – Takes up where Glow Nuture left off. Covers
  breastfeeding, sleep, feed and nap cycles.
- Start - Covers the monitoring, treatment and medication of
  depression. Helps to diagnose mental health problems and track
  the progress of treatments.

ResearchKit

What is ResearchKit?
ResearchKit is an open-source software framework created by Apple designed for medical and health professionals. Researchers and developers can use the software to build iPhone apps to gather medical data from volunteers around the world. That data can then be used in medical studies involving diabetes, cancer, cardiovascular disease, asthma and more. The apps developed using ResearchKit can also access data from the Apple HeathKit app – and the ability to gather all that data can become a valuable tool for medical research.

How does ResearchKit work?
The framework consists of a variety of customizable modules including a survey engine, a visual consent flow (a series of screens presenting the user with the explanation of what he or she is consenting to in using the app), and a group of tasks for the user to complete. The framework does not include a database module – developers need to provide their own data management system (making sure it meets the requirements for privacy and security).

How do you design a ResearchKit app?
The ResearchKit framework comes with two sample apps located in the samples folder: ORKSample and ORKCatalog. The ORKSample app demonstrates how to use the main features of ResearchKit — informed consent, surveys, active tasks, account creation, and passcode pin entry — and shows how to design a research app to ensure a satisfactory user experience. You can quickly prototype research ideas by modifying the sample app.

ORKSample has:
- Placeholder pages for providing a preview of the study
- A dashboard page for displaying results to participants
- A profile page that shows key user data as well as providing an easy-to-access link for withdrawing from a study
- An activities page that provides a list of all the study tasks

while ORKCatalog shows how to:
- Construct a task
- Present a task view controller
- Handle the delegate callbacks from the task view controller
- Access the structure of the results collected by the task

How do you setup a ResearchKit project?

There are a number of steps to setting up a ReseachKit project:

- Install Xcode – Xcode is the official IDE (Integrated Development Environment) for all Apple platforms. It's only available for OS X so you'll need a Mac in order to build a ResearchKit app – however, you won't need another device to test your app because Xcode has a built-in iPhone simulator.
- Create your app as an Xcode project. Xcode will keep track of all the source code, libraries, and other files associated with your app.
- Unless you want to code everything from scratch you can choose one of the project templates that Xcode provides, depending on the type of app you want to create.
- Enter some setup information (Product name, Organization name, programming language, device(s) the app will run on, etc.
- Download ResearchKit from GitHub.
- Configure your Xcode project to use ResearchKit as a "framework".
- Build your project app using the Xcode IDE.

The Future of Healthcare Apps

What's in store in the not-to-distant future for healthcare apps? Here are a couple of items that may be available soon:

- Injectable biosensors that can stream a person's medical data to smartphones (and the cloud) are being developed by researchers at Profusa. Current test results that the sensors have overcome the problems of local inflammation and scar tissue stemming from "foreign body response.
- University of Illinois researchers have developed a camera that could greatly improve the diagnostic capabilities of smartphones. The new camera can perform optical spectroscopy – fitted into a smartphone the technology could allow users to conduct tests normally done only a lab, such as identifying bio markers for cancer, sepsis, cardiac health, pregnancy, and infectious diseases. Then, by linking through the internet, the user could communicate in real time to clinicians and specialists.

Drawbacks to Healthcare Apps

The wave of healthcare and medical apps on the market promises benefits such as more responsive health care and more control over our own health and medical well-being. There is a downside however – as there is with any new technology. Concerns with the spread of healthcare apps include:
- The increased exposure of our private medical data to hackers or just to the public in general.
- A lessening of the face-to-face relationship between patient and doctor. Sometimes your doctor can catch potential problems simply because of his or her familiarity with you and your medical history.
- The increasing number of healthcare apps on the market that claim to be able to detect certain problems but fail to do so – or that notify you of a problem that doesn't really exist.
- Multiple agencies attempting to establish a regulatory system for mobile healthcare apps, creating a sometimes confusing (and expensive) landscape for mobile app developers.

Eventually these problems will be solved, but in the meantime be sure to do your due diligence when choosing a mobile healthcare app. The legitimate ones can go a long way toward helping you stay healthy.

Appendix A – Medical Terminology

ABC – Refers to checking Airways, Breathing and Circulation when administering resuscitation or life support.

Abduction - To move a limb or some other body part away from the midline of the body

ABG - arterial blood gas reading.

a.c.: Before meals. For example, taking your medicine before eating.

Acidotic - Abnormally high acidity of body fluids and tissues.

ACL: Anterior Cruciate Ligament; ACL injuries are one of the most common ligament injuries to the knee.

Acute – A sudden, severe condition as opposed to a long-term, chronic condition.

Acute Myocardial Infarction (heart attack) – Sudden damage to part of the heart muscle, usually due to blockage of the coronary arteries.

Adenoids - Small lumps of lymphatic tissue located at the back of the throat, above the tonsils. Together with the tonsils the adenoids are a part of the body's immune system, working to detect harmful bacteria and viruses. Both the adenoids and the tonsils can become infected and may need to be surgically removed.

Afebrile – Without fever; as opposed to febrile (feverish).

AIDS – Autoimmune Deficiency Syndrome.

AKA – An above the knee amputation.

Ambulant – Able to walk.

Anemia – A condition where there is a lack of red blood cells or of hemoglobin in the blood.

Angina – Cariac pain due to a poor blood supply to the heart.

Anoxia – Lack of oxygen.

Antibody – A substance produced by the immune system to fight invading organisms such as viruses.

Antioxidant - Any of numerous chemical substances including certain natural body products and nutrients that can neutralize the oxidant effect of free radicals and other substances. Free radicals, formed in the course of normal cellular respiration and metabolism, and more abundantly under the influence of certain environmental chemicals and sunlight, have been associated with various types of tissue damage, particularly those involved in atherosclerosis, the aging process, and the development of cancers.

Anuric - Not producing urine. Someone who is anuric is often critical and may need dialysis.

Aperient - A laxative.

Appendix - A tube-shaped sac attached protruding from the lower end of the large intestine; the exact function the appendix serves is still unknown. However, an inflamed appendix can be life-threatening if not treated promptly.

Appendicitis – Inflammation of the appendix, a finger-like projection of the colon.

Arthritis – Joint inflammation.

Asthma – A lung disease marked by difficulty in breathing and by chronic coughing.

Ataxia – A jerky unsteadiness of parts of the body due to disease centered in a particular part of the brain.

AutoImmune Deficiency Syndrome (AIDS) – A disease that involves a loss of immune system function.

Axial – Relating to the central part of the body as opposed to the limbs.

BCG – The Bacille Calmett-Guerin tuberculosis vaccination.

b.i.d. - Latin, bis a die, meaning twice daily; as in taking a certain medicine twice daily.

Bile - A bitter greenish-brown alkaline fluid secreted by the liver. Bile aids digestion and is stored in the gallbladder until it's released into the colon. (Note: People can live a reasonably normal life without a gall bladder).

Bibasilar - At the bases of both lungs. For example, someone with pneumonia in both lungs might have abnormal bibasilar breath sounds.

BKA – Below the knee amputation.

BMP: A basic metabolic panel, measuring the body's electrolytes (potassium, sodium, carbon dioxide, and chloride) as well as creatinine and glucose.

Body – The human body is composed of a number of different systems:
- Skeletal - Consists of 206 bones connected by tendons, ligaments and cartilage. The skeleton helps us move and is also involved in the production of blood cells and the storage of calcium. The teeth are also part of the skeletal system.
- Muscular – Muscles and tendons. Consists of approximately 650 muscles which are divided into three types: skeletal muscles which are connect to bone, smooth muscles found inside organs, and cardiac muscle found inside the heart. Skeletal muscles help us move, smooth muscle helps move substances through the organs, and cardiac muscle helps the heart pump blood through the body.
- Sensory - Eyes, ears, nose, skin receptors, and mouth.
- Integumentary – Consists of the skin (the largest organ in the body), hair, nails, and glands in the skin.
- Respiratory - Nose, pharynx, larynx, trachea, bronchi, and lungs.
- Cardiovascular (circulatory) - moves blood, nutrients, oxygen, carbon dioxide, and hormones around the body. It consists of the heart, blood, and blood vessels (arteries and veins).
- Gastrointestinal - Mouth, esophagus, stomach, small and large intestines, pancreas, liver, and gallbladder.

- Lymphatic (immune) - Tonsils, spleen, bone marrow, thymus, lymph nodes, lymphatic vessels, and lymph fluid.
- Endocrine - Consists of eight major glands that secrete hormones into the blood which, in turn, travel to different tissues and regulate different bodily functions such as metabolism, growth and sexual functions. The endocrine system includes the pituitary gland, thyroid, adrenal glands, hypothalamus, parathyroids, pineal gland, pancreas, and the reproductive glands.
- Reproductive - Ovaries, uterine tubes, uterus, and vagina in females; testes, ducts, penis, urethra, and prostate in males.
- Urinary - Kidneys, ureters, bladder, and urethra.
- Nervous - Brain, spinal cord, ganglia, nerves, and sensory organs.

BP – Blood pressure.

Bronchitis – Infection of the larger airways of the lungs.

BSO (Bilateral salpingo-oophorectomy) - The removal of both of the ovaries and the adjacent Fallopian tubes, often performed as part of a total abdominal hysterectomy.

Carotid arteries – Major blood vessels in the neck that supply blood to the brain, neck, and face. There are two carotid arteries, one on the right and one on the left side of the neck; they divide in the neck to form the external and internal carotid arteries.

CBC (Complete Blood Count) – Typically includes:
White blood cell count
Red blood cell count
Hematocrit (Hct)
Hemoglobin (Hbg)
Mean corpuscular volume (MCV)
Mean corpuscular hemoglobin (MCH)

Chem panel (Chemistry panel) - A blood test that indicates the status of the liver, kidneys, and electrolytes.

COPD (Chronic obstructive pulmonary disease) – A slowly progressive obstruction of airflow into and out of the lungs. COPD is usually caused by smoking or exposure to smoke, air pollution or an infectious disease.

CVA (Cerebrovascular accident) – A stroke.

D and C (Dilation and curettage) - Widening the cervix and scrapping with a curette to remove tissue lining the inner surface of the womb (uterus).

Digital Medicine – Generally defined as a combination of remote monitoring, behavior modification and personalized intervention involving the patient's own doctors.

DDX (Differential diagnosis) – Differentiating a particular disease or condition from others that share the same characteristics.

DM (Diabetes mellitus) - The most common form of diabetes, caused by a deficiency of the pancreatic hormone insulin, which results in a failure to metabolize sugars and starch.

DNR (Do not resuscitate) - A specific order not to revive a patient artificially. If a patient is given a DNR order, they aren't resuscitated if they are near death (no code blue is called).

Edema – Fluid retention in the body's tissues.

ePHI – Electronic Personal Health Information.

Esophagus – The part of the digestive tract between the mouth and the stomach.

FX – Fracture.

Gall bladder - A small organ where bile is stored and concentrated before it's released into the small intestine.

H&H (Hemoglobin and Hematocrit) – Low H&H indicates the presence of anemia. Elevated levels of H&H can indicate lung disease.

Haematoma – A well-defined bruise.

Haematuria – Blood in the urine.

Haemoglobin – An iron-containing protein found in red blood cells.

Haemoptysis – Coughing up blood.

Hepatitis – Inflammation of the liver, usually caused by viral infections such as Hepatitis C virus or by heavy alcohol use or other toxins. Hepatitis can be a static condition or it can progress to fibrosis, cirrhosis, or liver cancer.

Health Level 7 (H7) - Refers to a set of international standards for the transfer of clinical and administrative data between software applications used by various healthcare providers.

Hernia – An abnormal protrusion of the contents of one part of the body into another.

HTN (Hypertension) – Abnormally high blood pressure.

Hyperglycaemia – An elevated blood sugar level, often indicative of diabetes.

Hypertension – Above normal blood pressure.

Hypotension – Low blood pressure.

Insulin – A substance produced by the pancreas which is needed by the body to convert sugar to energy. Individuals suffering from diabetes lack sufficient insulin.

In vitro – In the laboratory.

Ischaemia – Lack of blood supply to some part of the body. Cardiac ischaemia for example may cause angina and in sever cases may trigger a heart attack.

Itegumentary system – The integumentary system is made up of the skin, hair, nails, and glands in the skin.

Kidneys – A pair of organs in the rear of the abdominal cavity; the kidneys regulate fluid balance in the body and filter out wastes from the blood in the form of urine.

Liver – The body's largest internal organ. Located in the upper right-hand portion of the abdominal cavity, the liver performs a variety of functions: produces proteins for blood plasma, stores & releases glucose as needed, produces bile to break down fats and carry away waste, processes hemoglobin and regulates blood clotting.

Lungs – Two large inflatable organs in the chest which remove oxygen from the air we breathe and transfer it to the arterial blood vessels to be sent to the rest of the body. The lungs also remove carbon dioxide from the veins so the carbon dioxide can be exhaled and eliminated from the body.

MMA – Mobile Medical Application

Mantoux test – A skin test used to help diagnose cases of tuberculosis.

Meningitis – Inflammation of the meninges, three protective membranes surrounding the brain.

Metacarpal fracture - A fracture of one of the five bones in the part of the hand between the wrist and the fingers.

Methylprednisolone - An anti-inflammatory steroid.

Morbidity – A description of the outcome of disease or the relative incidence of a particular disease in a certain locality.

MRI - Magnetic Resonance Imaging. Medical imaging by computer using a strong magnetic field and radio frequencies.

Munchausen Syndrome – A psychological condition where an individual lies about having a medical condition (or several different ones) in order to gain attention from medical personnel.

Myosis - Excessive contraction of the pupil in the eye.

Necrotic – Dead (tissue, etc.).

Neuritis – Inflammation of neural tissue.

NPO (nothing by mouth) – Latin, meaning nothing through the mouth. Withholding food and fluids from a patient for various reasons.

NS – Normal saline solution.

NSAID - Nonsteroid anti-inflammatory drug (such as Advil or Motrin).

Occipital – Back of the head.

Orbital fracture - A fracture of the bony socket that holds the eyeball.

Osteosarcoma - bone cancer.

Pancreas – A gland that lies behind the stomach and is responsible for producing insulin (which allows the body to convert sugar into energy).

Pancreatitis - Chronic or acute inflammation of the pancreas.

Paresis - Partial or slight paralysis.

Pathological – Related to a disease or abnormality.

Pediculosis – An infestation of the skin by the pediculosis louse (also known as scabies).

Peptic – Related to stomach acid, as in "peptic ulcer".

Pericardium - The sac that covers the heart.

Phlebitis – Inflammation of a vein.

Platelets (thrombocytes) - A component of blood whose function (along with the coagulation factors) is to stop bleeding by clumping together and clotting blood vessel injuries. If your blood is low in platelets, it's a condition called thrombocytopenia which can put you at risk for mild to serious bleeding. If your blood has too many platelets, you may have a higher risk of blood clots.

Pleura - the lining around the lung.

Pneumothorax – A condition where air leaks into the space between the chest wall and a lung causing the lung to uncouple itself from the chest wall. A pneumothorax is also referred to as "collapsed lung".

Ptosis - Drooping of the eyelid.

Pulmonary edema - Fluid in the lungs.

Pulmonary embolus – A condition where an embolus (blood clot) lodges in the lung tissue.

Pulse rate – The number of heart beats per minute measured from a pulsating artery (normally about 70 beatstimes per minute.

Pyelogram - An x-ray of the kidneys using an intravenously inserted dye.

Rapid infuser - A device that transports blood into the system at a fast rate to help prevent hypohemia.

Reflux - Moving backward in the esophagus.

Renogram - An x-ray of the kidneys.

Rifampin - An antibiotic used to treat tuberculosis, meningitis, leprosy, and staph infections.

Ringer's solution - An intravenous solution consisting of salt, potassium, and calcium boiled in water used to counteract dehydration.

Sepsis - A very severe infection.

Spleen – An organ in the upper left abdominal area which is part of the body's immune system. The spleen acts as a filter for blood; old red blood cells are recycled in the spleen, and platelets and white blood cells are stored there.

Splenectomy - Surgical removal of the spleen.

Stasis - Slowing or stopping of blood flow.

Stat – Immediately.

Tachycardia – An extremely rapid heart beat with a pulse rate of over 100 beats per minute.

Tetanus – A serious bacterial infection which begins in uncleaned wounds and can lead to paralysis.

Tension pneumothorax - A collapsed lung.

Thiamine (Vitamin B1) – An important vitamin needed for the brain and heart.

Thoracic – Pertains to the chest.

Thoracotomy - Surgery on the thoracic area (chest cavity).

Thrombosis - A blood clot.

Tonsils - Two small masses of lymphoid tissue in the throat, one on each side of the root of the tongue. Tonsils (along with the adenoids) are a part of the body's immune system – they trap germs entering the body through the mouth or nose.

Trachea (windpipe)   A large membranous tube reinforced by rings of cartilage, extending from the larynx to the bronchial tubes. The trachea carries air to and from the lungs.

Tuberculosis – A serious bacterial infection of the lungs (or on occasion, the kidneys).

URI (Upper Respiratory Infection) - An acute infection involving the upper respiratory tract including the nose, sinuses, pharynx or larynx. The different types of upper respiratory infection include tonsillitis, pharyngitis, laryngitis, sinusitis, otitis media, and the common cold.

Uric acid - An acid formed when nucleoproteins are broken down in tissues. A person's uric acid is often tested when gout is suspected since a high uric acid content in the blood often causes gout symptoms and the formation of stones.

Urological – Pertaining to the bladder, kidneys or urinary system.

V-fib - Ventricular fibrillation.

Venipuncture - Drawing of blood from a vein.

Virus – An infectious agent about 100 times smaller than a bacteria cell. It only reproduces inside of a host cell and can infect both animals and plants.

WBC – White blood cell count.

Appendix B – Useful Resources

https://mhealthintelligence.com/ - Articles, interviews, webcasts and news of upcoming events concerning mobile healthcare and medical apps.

https://imedicalapps.com - iMedicalApps is one of the leading online publications for medical professionals, patients, and anyone interested in mobile medical technology and health care apps. The website publishes reviews, research, and commentary on mobile medical technology from physicians, medical personnel and other healthcare professionals.

https://www.fda.gov/medicaldevices/digitalhealth/mobileme dicalapplications/default.htm – Information on FDA regulation of mobile medical applications.

https://www.raywenderlich.com/929-carekit-tutorial-for-ios-part-1 – Brief CareKit tutorial showing how to use CareKit to actually build an app that helps people to manage their medical conditions.

https://thinkmobiles.com/blog/how-to-make-healthcare-app - Develops healthcare apps (note: you can share the cost with others who want basically the same app).

Https://www.appypie.com – mobile app builder (make an app without coding).

Https://www.mobilesmith.com – Offers mobile app packages for hospitals and other healthcare organizations. Packages include one that has apps that address hospital access and pregnancy and another one that has apps that deal with general and special surgeries.

https://www.modolabs.com/products-youll-love-2/hospital-apps/ - ModoLabs' *Modo Workplace for Hospitals* system is designed to allow hospitals and medical centers to quickly create apps for patients, employees and visitors.   Apps can be created by integrating existing data sources with pre-built modules like Patient Education, Tour, dining, news and maps.

https://medcitynews.com/tag/mobile-health-news/ - Covers the mobile healthcare app market with articles ranging from which business plan for marketing mobile medical apps seems to be working the best to the FDA clearing an ultrasound app for pregnant women.

https://www.pepperlaw.com/resource/22623/18D3 – An article entitled "Where's the App for That? Mobile Medical Apps, Cybersecurity and the Regulatory and Litigation Landscape" that covers many of the problems involved in creating a mobile medical app that meets the requirements of various regulatory agencies.

https://forums.studentdoctor.net/forums/tech-medical-apps-ios-android-medical-devices.109/ - Healthcare and medical app forums.

http://researchkit.org/docs/docs/Overview/GuideOverview.html – ResearchKit Framework Programming Guide (includes an overview of the ResearchKit framework and a detailed explanation of each of the ResearchKit modules).

https://www.altova.com/mobile-development-tool - MobileTogether is a mobile development framework for building data-centric apps for any device. Note: According to the website Mobile Together Designer is free to use – just download and ask for a free key code to unlock the software.

https://www.mobihealthnews.com/ - Articles on mobile healthcare events, devices, apps and news in general.

Appendix C – Creating a Secure Medical App

Thanks to advances in mobile technology smartphone users can now access and share their medical records right on their phone. With great access though comes great responsibility. The importance of keeping personal medical information private means that securing that information is a vital part of any mobile medical app.

If you're creating your app yourself (or even if you're having someone else do it), be sure to find out what agency or agencies have regulations your app has to comply with and what those regulations cover. Organizations that may have a say about your app include the FDA, the Department of Commerce, the FTC, and the Office for Civil Rights among others. Regardless of who is involved you will need to meet the privacy requirements of each agency by integrating security features into your app such as:
- Encrypting any eHealth data stored on the user's phone.
- Requiring users to log in using multi-factor authentication (such as a login name and password plus a single-use authentication code).
- Add cybersecurity routines to your app (be sure to read the FDA's 2016 draft guidance that identifies steps mobile medical app producers should take to identify and address cybersecurity vulnerabilities that pose a risk to patient safety and public health).
- Carry out extensive security testing to identify any weaknesses in your security routines. Areas of concern include:
  - Inadequate user authorization and authentication
  - Insecure data storage (sensitive data is being stored with insufficient file permissions that leave it vulnerable to unauthorized access)
  - Inadequate encryption algorithms
  - Client-side injection attacks (the app doesn't check input closely enough leaving user data at risk)
  - Inadequate transport layer protection (the communication channel between the app and the server isn't secure)
  - Insufficient protection of the app binary code leaving it open \to hi-jacking
  - Data leakage (eHealth data stored on the device isn't properly insulated from other apps)

- Plan for future updates to keep pace with new security threats.
- Conduct extensive "beta" tests with a small group of users once the app is compiled in order to catch any security holes that weren't uncovered in pre-release testing.

Appendix D – Medical Devices and Smartphones

Medical apps are making use of the sensors built into your smartphone as well as a growing number of medical devices that are designed to work with your smartphone or other mobile device. Here a just a few of the apps utilizing built-in or add-on sensors:

- Liftpulse – Uses the iPhone's accelerometer to measure tremt a ors in patients suffering from Parkinson's Disease.
- Apple's Medical ID turns any iPhone 4s or later into a mobile medical alert bracelet. Setting the Medical ID on your phone allows emergency personnel to tap and hold the Emergency button on your home screen (even if the phone's locked) to get access to your medical condition(s), emergency contacts, allergies, blood type and other data.
- Ihealth Lab's Wireless Smart Gluco-Monitoring System is an FDA approved glucometer that measures the glucose levels in your blood and displays the data on your smartphone.
- 6SenSor Lab's portable gluten detector is designed to work with their app that allows you to track and share data with others.
- AliveCor's FDA approved EKG monitor, coupled with their dedicated app delivers a medical-grade electrocardiogram (ECG) to your smartphone within 30 seconds.
- Alcohoot, a mobile breathalyzer connects with your smartphone to display your blood alcohol level.
- HemaApp uses your smartphone's camera to screen for anemia.
- Biliscreen can help screen for cancer and other diseases by analyzing the schlera or white part of the eye in selfies.
- Propeller Health has developed "smart" inhalers with can communicate with smartphones via Bluetooth.
- AsthmaMD is a small portable flow meter used to gauge lung performance. It works with an accompanying app that allows the user to keep a detailed record of asthma attacks and pass that data on to a physician or other medical personnel.
- Cardiio uses your smartphone camera to detect facial signs of a heart arrhythmia associated with strokes. It works by measuring and analyzing tiny changes of light reflected on the skin as the result of the underlying pulse.

And many others are being added every day as the smartphone becomes more and more important to healthcare.

Appendix E – Mini Med School

There are a growing number of mobile medical apps for medical school students, including some very sophisticated ones. Here are a few of the top-rated apps which, taken as a group, could almost serve as a mini medical school on their own:

Lexicomp
With databases for drug information and interactions, dosing, OTCs and natural products, lab and diagnostic procedures, toxicology, and even dental, Lexicomp provides comprehensive reference information. The service is subscription-based, and can be expensive, but institutions often have subscriptions and database access can be purchased one item at a time.

Ward Round
Developed by Guerilla Tea, Ward Round (for iOS) offers an entertaining game-based way to test your readiness for clinical rounds. You're presented with a quick case simulation drawn from one of nine different medical specialties and asked to answer a series of questions pertaining to that case. You then have 12 seconds to analyze the clinical information and come up with the correct clinical answer to each question. Once you submit your answer you get immediate feedback on which answer was correct and why. At the end of each case you're given a percentage rating based on the number of questions you answered correctly. The medical specialties covered are Cardiology, Endocrinology, Gastrointestinal, Hematology-Oncology, Infectious Diseases, Musculoskeletal, Neurology, Renal/Genitourinary, and Respiratory.

Essential Anatomy 5
This app lets you view any body system, rotate it in any direction, zoom in and out, hide and reveal structures as desired, and tap on individual structures to have them identified and explained. Muscles can be added and subtracted in multiple layers. You can also add bookmarks; search for anatomical structures by name; scribble on any part of the model in glowing green pencil to call attention to details of interest; share a particular view with friends and associates in any number of ways; and take quizzes to evaluate your anatomical knowledge.

Prognosis

Prognosis is a free app that allows you to test your diagnostic ability with over 600 simulated clinical case scenarios (with new ones added weekly). Each case has a short, in-depth analysis of the diagnostic process, followed by an up-to-date discussion on the specific condition involved. The cases cover over 30 specialties and each one is reviewed by volunteer specialists who make sure that each scenario is accurate and clinically relevant.

Anatomy & Physiology in a Flash!

This multi-media app from the Skyscape provides reference information and flashcards for anyone looking to develop a basic understanding of the functions and structures of the human body. It includes 15 sections organized by body system and color-coded and each section contains tips and quiz questions to test the user's understanding of the material in that section. There are over 250 full color flash cards covering the body's structures and the cards can be bookmarked for additional study later. Users can also create custom quizzes to improve areas of weakness based on answered questions. The app also provides a question of the day . Note: In-app purchases must be made in order to access all questions.

Diseases Dictionary Medical

This free medical dictionary and thesaurus app is great for students and healthcare professionals alike since it can be downloaded for offline access. It provides comprehensive information about medical conditions, diseases, symptoms, causes, treatment, prescription drugs, interactions, side effects, etc.

Drugs Dictionary

free pharmaceuticals dictionary app that can be accessed offline, with a user-friendly interface and detailed information about a huge range of drugs. It includes everything from drug uses and dosage to interactions, side effects, precautions, storage instructions, missed dosages and more.

MedCalX

Like other medical apps for medical students and professionals, this easy-to-use calculator helps you save time and make faster decisions in critical situations. The app gives you instant access a huge variety of medical calculations, including scores, formulas, classifications and scales, as well as your own most-used equations.

Radiology 2.0

CT scans take a great deal of training to read correctly, which is why many medical students spend hours staring at screens, referencing books, and trying to figure out what they are seeing. Radiology 2.0 aims to help with this by providing an interactive education in radiology. Extensive discussions follow each case to explain what you are seeing and the meaning behind it. This app uses many images (over 7,000!) to help you learn to interpret CT scans correctly.

Touch Surgery

Touch Surgery (free for iOS and Android) is an interactive surgical simulator that guides you through a variety of operations. You can:
- Learn operations step-by-step in training mode
- Experience realistic surgical environments with state of the art 3D graphics
- Track your results as a surgeon
- Build a personalized library of surgical procedures
- Learn new techniques
- Use the spy glass feature to identify and learn about the instruments, tissues, muscles and bones involved in each procedure

iSurf Brain View

This app uses neuroimaging information based on T1 MRI images to help you learn about the brain MRI field and neuroanatomy in general. Automatic segmentation helps to produce an atlas of neuroimages for the student to study. Tools let you zoom in, identify structures, make notes, and more.

3M Littman SoundBuilder

Littman is a 3M-owned company that creates medical-grade stethoscopes, and the SoundBuilder app has the same purpose (albeit with an educational twist): improving the auscultation skills of students and practicing clinicians. 14 lessons provide an education in key heart sounds using text, a virtual mannequin, dynamic waveforms, and a 3D animation of a heart in action. Headphones are definitely recommended, since the difference between a healthy heart and a problematic one can be hard to pin down.

Clearpath

Clearpath deals with dermatopathology (the study and diagnosis of diseases of the skin and associated mucous membranes). It provides you with a fully searchable, comprehensive pictorial atlas of skin lesions. Multiple examples are provided for each type, and a virtual microscope enables you to zoom in on select images to view them at various magnifications. In test mode, you're confronted with random slides and asked to choose which of a long list of diagnoses they exemplify. These images can also be zoomed in on to view them in greater detail. For an extra challenge, a limited amount of time is allotted to respond to each slide. Note: Clearpath is only available for Apple devices.